YOUR KNOWLEDGE HAS VALUE

Evaluation of different Analytic Tools for promoting Evidence-Based Public Health

Awung Nkeze Elvis

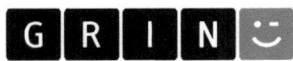

Bibliographic information published by the German National Library:

The German National Library lists this publication in the National Bibliography; detailed bibliographic data are available on the Internet at http://dnb.dnb.de.

ISBN: 9783346929723
This book is also available as an ebook.

© GRIN Publishing GmbH
Trappentreustraße 1
80339 München

Print and binding: Books on Demand GmbH, Norderstedt, Germany
Printed on acid-free paper from responsible sources.

The present work has been carefully prepared. Nevertheless, authors and publishers do not incur liability for the correctness of information, notes, links and advice as well as any printing errors.

GRIN web shop: https://www.grin.com/document/1382446

Title: Exploring the effectiveness of analytic tools for promoting evidence-based public health

Subtitle: Evaluation of Different Analytic Tools for Promoting Evidence-Based Public Health

By

Awung Nkeze Elvis

ABSTRACT

Evidence-based public health is a concept that emphasizes the use of scientific evidence in decision-making processes related to public health. To promote the uptake of EBPH, various analytic tools can be employed. Systematic reviews and economic evaluations can be used to help promote evidence-based practices. This study explores the effectiveness of different analytic tools in promoting EBPH. Randomised controlled trials (RCTs), which are the gold standard in evidence-based medicine when it comes to public health, may not always be practical or appropriate for evaluating public health initiatives (Kemm, 2006). The complexity of public health initiatives, which frequently target communities rather than individuals, as well as the significance of context and social determinants of health, must be taken into consideration (Kemm, 2006). To integrate many evidence sources and handle the complexity of public health, other methodologies and analytical tools are required. Although these tools provide insightful information for practitioners and policymakers, they still require improvement in order to address complicated public health issues and incorporate a variety of evidence sources.

Keywords: Public Health, evidence-based public health, effectiveness of analytic tools, scientific evidence

INTRODUCTION

The essential idea of "evidence-based public health" (EBPH) emphasises the use of the best available scientific information in public health decision-making processes (Brownson et al., 2009). It entails making decisions based on thorough research, adopting program-planning frameworks, using data and information systems methodically, including the community in decision-making, carrying out reliable evaluations, and communicating the results (Brownson et al., 2009). In order to ensure that public health initiatives are successful and supported by strong evidence, EBPH aims to close the gap between research and practise (Brownson et al., 2009). Various analytical tools can be used to encourage the adoption of EBPH. One such instrument that helps hasten the adoption of evidence-based practises is systematic reviews (Fielding, 2009). Systematic reviews involve a comprehensive and rigorous synthesis of existing research evidence on a specific topic. They provide a summary of the available evidence, evaluate its quality, and draw conclusions based on the collective findings of multiple studies (Fielding, 2009). By synthesizing the evidence in a systematic and transparent manner, systematic reviews help inform decision-making processes and guide the implementation of evidence-based interventions (Fielding, 2009). Economic evaluations are another important analytic tool in promoting the uptake of EBPH. Economic evaluations assess the costs and benefits of different interventions, allowing decision-makers to prioritize resources and allocate them effectively (Terris-Prestholt et al., 2016). By considering the economic implications of implementing evidence-based interventions, economic evaluations provide valuable information on the cost-effectiveness and affordability of public health programs (Terris-Prestholt et al., 2016).

This knowledge can impact policy choices and aid in the adoption of solutions that provide the most financial value (Terris-Prestholt et al., 2016). Other techniques that assist the adoption of an evidence-based strategy in public health practise have been created in addition to systematic reviews and economic evaluations. These resources for planning and training include grey literature, policy tracking and surveillance tools, health surveillance systems, and evidence-based guidelines (Jacobs et al., 2012). According to Jacobs et al. (2012), each of these instruments has a particular function in promoting the adoption of EBPH, such as offering advice on programme development, data gathering, and assessment. To enhance the effectiveness of these analytic tools, it is important to build capacity for evidence-based public health. Capacity building involves providing the necessary resources, structures, and workforce to plan, deliver, and evaluate evidence-based interventions (Brownson et al., 2018). This can be achieved through various approaches, such as technical assistance, knowledge brokering, assessment and feedback, and peer networking (Brownson et al., 2018). These approaches aim to enhance the skills and knowledge of public health practitioners, promote the use of EBPH in organizational settings, and foster collaboration and knowledge exchange among practitioners (Brownson et al., 2018).

In conclusion, the effectiveness of different analytic tools, including systematic reviews and economic evaluations, in promoting the uptake of EBPH is well-established. These tools provide valuable evidence and information that can inform decision-making processes, guide the implementation of evidence-based interventions, and prioritize resources effectively. However, it is important to also consider other tools and approaches, such as capacity building and knowledge exchange, to ensure the successful adoption and implementation of EBPH in public health practice.

General Objective:

The general objective of this study is to explore the effectiveness of different analytic tools, such as systematic reviews and economic evaluations, in promoting the uptake of evidence-based public health (EBPH).

Specific Objectives:

1. To describe and evaluate the quality of economic evaluations of clinical pharmacy services (CPS) published between 2006 and 2010, with the goal of informing administrators and practitioners about their cost-effectiveness (Touchette et al., 2014).

2. To identify and analyze studies that evaluate CPS and describe economic and clinical outcomes, including methodology used, economic evaluation type, CPS setting and type, and clinical and economic outcome results (Touchette et al., 2014).

3. To assess the impact of CPS on clinical, economic, and humanistic outcomes in various settings, such as hospitals, community pharmacies, and ambulatory practices (Touchette et al., 2014).

4. To determine the presence of control groups and the justification of study assumptions and limitations in economic evaluations of CPS (Touchette et al., 2014).

5. To calculate and report benefit-cost ratios and incremental cost-effectiveness ratios in economic evaluations of CPS (Touchette et al., 2014).

6. To examine the relationship between the effectiveness of systematic reviews and economic evaluations and the uptake of EBPH in decision-making processes (Fielding, 2009).

7. To identify common CPS settings, such as hospitals, community pharmacies, and clinic or hospital-based ambulatory practices, and the types of CPS evaluated, including disease state

management, general pharmacotherapeutic monitoring, target drug programs, and patient education (Touchette et al., 2014).

DISCUSSION AND IMPLICATIONS

Quality of economic evaluations of clinical pharmacy services (CPS) published between 2006 and 2010 Touchette et al. (2014) were previously evaluated in three systematic reviews conducted by (Touchette et al., 2014). The objective of these reviews was to assess the cost-effectiveness of CPS and provide information to administrators and practitioners. In these systematic reviews, identified and analyzed studies that evaluated CPS and described their economic and clinical outcomes (Touchette et al., 2014). The methodology used in these economic evaluations, including the type of economic evaluation, the setting and type of CPS, and the results of both clinical and economic outcomes, were assessed (Touchette et al., 2014). One important aspect of evaluating the quality of economic evaluations is the presence of control groups and the justification of study assumptions and limitations (Touchette et al., 2014). By examining these factors, were able to assess the robustness and reliability of the economic evaluations of CPS. Furthermore, benefit-cost ratios and incremental cost-effectiveness ratios were calculated and reported in these economic evaluations (Touchette et al., 2014). These ratios provide valuable information on the cost-effectiveness of CPS interventions and assist decision-makers in resource allocation. Overall, the systematic reviews conducted by aimed to comprehensively evaluate the quality of economic evaluations of CPS published between 2006 and 2010. The synthesis of available evidence aimed to inform administrators and practitioners about the cost-effectiveness of CPS and support evidence-based decision-making in healthcare settings. To identify and analyze studies that evaluate CPS and describe economic and clinical outcomes, including methodology used, economic evaluation type, CPS setting and type, and clinical and economic outcome results, several references can be used. References Husereau et al. (2013), provide information on economic evaluations and their importance in decision-making and health technology assessment. These references emphasise the requirement for reporting guidelines in economic evaluations as well as the difficulties in disclosing the expenses and effects of health interventions. Reference The Consolidated Health Economic Evaluation Reporting Standards (CHEERS) statement, which intends to offer instructions for reporting economic evaluations, is especially covered by Husereau et al. (2013). In economic evaluations, the authors stress the significance of reporting resource consumption, expenditures, preference-related data, and cost-effectiveness results. References The emphasis of Brownson et al. (2009) is on evidence-based public health (EBPH) and the difficulties in implementing and disseminating it. Despite the fact that these references are not specifically related to economic analyses of CPS, they offer insights into the larger context of evidence-based practises and the obstacles to their adoption in public health practise. It is advised to conduct a systematic literature review using pertinent databases like Medline, International Pharmaceutical Abstracts, Embase, and Cumulative Index to Nursing and Allied Health Literature in order to specifically identify studies that evaluate CPS and describe economic and clinical outcomes. The search strategy should include keywords related to CPS, economic evaluation, clinical outcomes, and methodology. The inclusion criteria should specify the publication period between 2006 and 2010. Once the relevant studies are identified, a thorough analysis can be conducted to extract information on the methodology used, economic evaluation type (e.g., cost-effectiveness analysis, cost-utility analysis), CPS setting and type, and the results of both clinical and economic outcomes. The economic evaluations of CPS within the chosen time period will be thoroughly explained, along with their implications for cost-effectiveness and healthcare decision-making. Numerous studies have evaluated the effect of Clinical Pharmacy Services (CPS) on clinical, financial, and humanistic outcomes in a range of contexts, including hospitals, community pharmacies, and ambulatory practises. Australia's community pharmacy diabetic service approach was the subject of research by Krass et al. in 2007. They discovered that the strategy produced considerable improvements in clinical and psychosocial outcomes for Type 2 diabetic patients. The study emphasised the role community chemists play in enhancing diabetes patients' care and overall health. A comprehensive review was carried out by Schumock et al. in 2003 to evaluate the financial effects of clinical pharmacy services. They discovered that the reviews' investigations concentrated on numerous practise settings, such as hospitals, neighbourhood pharmacies, clinics, and long-term care facilities. The clinical pharmacy services that were examined included everything from standard pharmacotherapeutic monitoring to patient education and disease management initiatives. The majority of research found that the clinical pharmacy services examined had positive financial effects. According to the review by Schumock et al. (2003), the economic benefits of clinical pharmacy services outweighed the expenses associated with providing those services. More than $4 in benefits were anticipated for every $1 spent on clinical pharmacy services. The studies' claimed benefit-cost ratios ranged from 1.7:1 to 17.0:1.In conclusion, the research by Krass et al. (2007) and Schumock et al. (2003) shows that CPS has a favourable effect on clinical, financial, and humanistic results. These findings support the role of pharmacists in improving patient care and health outcomes in various healthcare settings. To determine the presence of control groups and the justification of study assumptions and limitations in economic evaluations of Clinical Pharmacy Services (CPS), the systematic review conducted by Touchette et al. (2014) provides relevant information. In this review, the authors assessed the economic evaluations of CPS published between 2006 and 2010. According to (Touchette et al., 2014), control groups were included in 16 out of 23 studies that did not involve modeling. This suggests that the majority of the reviews' research used control groups to assess the effects of CPS interventions with a standard care or control group. According to Touchette et al. (2014)'s research on the justification of study assumptions and limits, eight studies (32%) explicitly expressed and defended their premises. This shows that a sizable majority of the CPS economic evaluations reported the study's assumptions and limitations in a transparent manner. According to the results of this systematic review, control groups were frequently utilised in economic analyses of CPS, and a sizable number of research offered reasons for their presumptions and limits. These procedures improve the economic assessments' validity and dependability and raise the studies' general standard of excellence. To calculate and report benefit-cost ratios and incremental cost-effectiveness ratios in economic evaluations of Clinical Pharmacy Services (CPS), the systematic review conducted by Touchette et al. (2014) provides relevant information. In this review, the authors assessed the economic evaluations of CPS published between 2006 and 2010. Touchette et al. (2014) reported that benefit-cost ratios were reported in three studies included in the review. The ratios ranged from 1.05:1 to 25.95:1, indicating that the benefits of CPS outweighed the costs in these studies. Additionally, five studies included in the review calculated and reported incremental cost-effectiveness ratios. However, specific details regarding the ratios were not provided in the reference. These findings suggest that benefit-cost ratios and incremental cost-effectiveness ratios were reported in a subset of the economic evaluations of CPS included in the review. The benefit-cost ratios indicated the economic value of CPS interventions, while the incremental cost-effectiveness ratios provided insights into the additional costs required to achieve specific health outcomes. It is important to note that the specific values of the benefit-cost ratios and incremental cost-effectiveness ratios may vary depending on the context, intervention, and study design. Therefore, it is recommended to refer to the original studies identified in the systematic review by Touchette et al. (2014) for more detailed information on the specific ratios reported. The relationship between the effectiveness of systematic reviews and economic evaluations and the uptake of Evidence-Based Public Health (EBPH) in decision-making processes has been explored in the literature. Brownson et al. (2009) discuss the role of analytic tools, including systematic reviews and economic evaluations, in accelerating the uptake of EBPH. They highlight the challenges and opportunities associated with disseminating EBPH, including political issues and training needs. Anderson (2009) questions the value of conducting systematic reviews of economic evaluations to inform decision-making in healthcare. The author argues that the wide range of factors that limit the generalizability of cost-effectiveness results and the context-dependency of resource use and opportunity costs undermine the value of systematic reviews of economic evaluations. On the other hand, Mastrigt et al. (2016) emphasize the importance of systematic reviews of economic evaluations in synthesizing economic evidence about health interventions. They highlight the methodological rigor of systematic reviews and their usefulness in informing evidence-based healthcare decisions. The systematic review by Luhnen et al. (2017) focuses on the characteristics and methods applied in systematic reviews of health economic evaluations. The study aims to analyze the methods used in systematic reviews of economic evaluations and identify common challenges. Overall, the literature provides differing perspectives on the utility and value of systematic reviews of economic evaluations in informing decision-making processes in healthcare. While some argue for their importance in synthesizing economic evidence, others highlight the challenges and limitations associated with generalizability and context-dependency. Based on the provided references, common Clinical Pharmacy Services (CPS) settings and types of CPS evaluated can be identified as follows:

Common CPS Settings:

1. Hospitals: Several studies reported evaluations of CPS in hospital settings (Perez et al., 2009; Touchette et al., 2014; Talon et al., 2019).

2. Community Pharmacies: Evaluations of CPS were also conducted in community pharmacy settings (Perez et al., 2009; Touchette et al., 2014; Talon et al., 2019).

3. Ambulatory Care Clinics or Physician's Offices: CPS evaluations were performed in ambulatory care settings (Perez et al., 2009; Talon et al., 2019).

Types of CPS Evaluated:

1. Disease State Management: Disease state management services were commonly evaluated in CPS studies (Perez et al., 2009; Touchette et al., 2014; Talon et al., 2019).

2. General Pharmacotherapeutic Monitoring: General pharmacotherapeutic monitoring services were frequently assessed in CPS evaluations (Perez et al., 2009; Touchette et al., 2014; Talon et al., 2019).

3. Target Drug Programs: Some studies focused on evaluating CPS related to target drug programs (Perez et al., 2009; Touchette et al., 2014; Talon et al., 2019).

4. Patient Education: Patient education services provided by CPS were also evaluated in certain studies (Perez et al., 2009; Talon et al., 2019).

It is important to note that the references provided cover different time periods, ranging from 2001 to 2017. Therefore, the distribution of CPS settings and types may vary across different time periods and regions. Additionally, the references provide insights into the economic evaluations of CPS and their impact, which can further inform decision-making processes in healthcare. These specific objectives aim to provide a comprehensive understanding of the effectiveness of analytic tools, such as systematic reviews and economic evaluations, in promoting the uptake of EBPH. By evaluating the quality and outcomes of economic evaluations of CPS and analyzing their impact in different settings, this study will contribute to the evidence base for decision-making in public health practice. Reference Touchette et al. (2014): , "Economic Evaluations of Clinical Pharmacy Services: 2006-2010," Pharmacotherapy: The Journal of Human Pharmacology and Drug Therapy (2014). doi:10.1002/phar.1414

CONCLUSION

Evidence-Based Public Health (EBPH) is an approach that aims to improve the scientific standards and generate well-grounded evidence in order to improve the health of the target population (Vanagas et al., 2017). In order to promote the adoption of EBPH, it is important to explore the effectiveness of different analytic tools, such as systematic reviews and economic evaluations (Kemm, 2006). Systematic reviews are a commonly used analytic tool in public health research. They involve a rigorous and transparent process of identifying, appraising, and synthesizing all available evidence on a specific topic (Atkinson et al., 2015). Systematic reviews provide a comprehensive and unbiased summary of the existing evidence, allowing policymakers and practitioners to make informed decisions based on the best available evidence (Atkinson et al., 2015). Economic evaluations are another important analytic tool in public health. They assess the costs and benefits of different interventions or policies, helping policymakers prioritize resources and make efficient and effective decisions (Atkinson et al., 2015). Economic evaluations can provide valuable information on the cost-effectiveness and cost-benefit of interventions, which is crucial for resource allocation in public health (Atkinson et al., 2015). The limitations of these analytical tools must be understood, though. Randomised controlled trials (RCTs), which are the gold standard in evidence-based medicine when it comes to public health, may not always be practical or appropriate for evaluating public health initiatives (Kemm, 2006). The complexity of public health initiatives, which frequently target communities rather than individuals, as well as the significance of context and social determinants of health, must be taken into consideration (Kemm, 2006). Therefore, alternative approaches and analytic tools that can integrate diverse evidence sources and consider the complexity of public health problems are needed (Atkinson et al., 2015).

In conclusion, exploring the effectiveness of different analytic tools, such as systematic reviews and economic evaluations, is crucial for promoting the adoption of Evidence-Based Public Health. While these tools have their limitations, they provide valuable insights and evidence for policymakers and practitioners to make informed decisions and design effective interventions and policies (Kemm, 2006; Atkinson et al., 2015). However, it is important to continue developing and refining analytic tools that can address the complexity of public health problems and integrate diverse evidence sources (Atkinson et al., 2015).

REFERENCES

Anderson, R. (2009, April 20). Systematic reviews of economic evaluations: utility or futility? *Health Economics*, *19*(3), 350–364. https://doi.org/10.1002/hec.1486

Atkinson, J. A., Page, A., Wells, R., Milat, A., & Wilson, A. (2015, March 3). A modelling tool for policy analysis to support the design of efficient and effective policy responses for complex public health problems. *Implementation Science*, *10*(1). https://doi.org/10.1186/s13012-015-0221-5

Brownson, R. C., Fielding, J. E., & Green, L. W. (2018, April 1). Building Capacity for Evidence-Based Public Health: Reconciling the Pulls of Practice and the Push of Research. *Annual Review of Public Health*, *39*(1), 27–53. https://doi.org/10.1146/annurev-publhealth-040617-014746

Brownson, R. C., Fielding, J. E., & Maylahn, C. M. (2009, April 1). Evidence-Based Public Health: A Fundamental Concept for Public Health Practice. *Annual Review of Public Health*, *30*(1), 175–201. https://doi.org/10.1146/annurev.publhealth.031308.100134

Brownson, R. C., Fielding, J. E., & Maylahn, C. M. (2009, April 1). Evidence-Based Public Health: A Fundamental Concept for Public Health Practice. *Annual Review of Public Health*, *30*(1), 175–201. https://doi.org/10.1146/annurev.publhealth.031308.100134

Fielding, J. E. (2009, April 1). Preface. *Annual Review of Public Health*, *30*(1). https://doi.org/10.1146/annurev.pu.30.031709.100001

Husereau, D., Drummond, M., Petrou, S., Carswell, C., Moher, D., Greenberg, D., Augustovski, F., Briggs, A. H., Mauskopf, J., & Loder, E. (2013, March 26). Consolidated Health Economic Evaluation Reporting Standards (CHEERS) Statement. *PharmacoEconomics*, *31*(5), 361–367. https://doi.org/10.1007/s40273-013-0032-y

Jacobs, J., Jones, E., Gabella, B., Spring, B., & Brownson, R. (2012, June). Tools for Implementing an Evidence-Based Approach in Public Health Practice. *Preventing Chronic Disease*. https://doi.org/10.5888/pcd9.110324

Kemm, J. (2006, May 22). The limitations of 'evidence-based' public health. *Journal of Evaluation in Clinical Practice*, *12*(3), 319–324. https://doi.org/10.1111/j.1365-2753.2006.00600.x

Krass, I., Armour, C. L., Mitchell, B., Brillant, M., Dienaar, R., Hughes, J., Lau, P., Peterson, G., Stewart, K., Taylor, S., & Wilkinson, J. (2007, June). The Pharmacy Diabetes Care Program: assessment of a community pharmacy diabetes service model in Australia. *Diabetic Medicine*, *24*(6), 677–683. https://doi.org/10.1111/j.1464-5491.2007.02143.x

Luhnen, M., Prediger, B., Neugebauer, E. A. M., & Mathes, T. (2017, December). Systematic reviews of health economic evaluations: a protocol for a systematic review of characteristics and methods applied. *Systematic Reviews*, *6*(1). https://doi.org/10.1186/s13643-017-0639-8

Perez, A., Doloresco, F., Hoffman, J. M., Meek, P. D., Touchette, D. R., Vermeulen, L. C., & Schumock, G. T. (2009, January). Economic Evaluations of Clinical Pharmacy Services: 2001–2005. *Pharmacotherapy*, *29*(1), 128–128. https://doi.org/10.1592/phco.29.1.128

Schumock, G. T., Butler, M. G., Meek, P. D., Vermeulen, L. C., Arondekar, B. V., & Bauman, J. L. (2003, January). Evidence of the Economic Benefit of Clinical Pharmacy Services: 1996–2000. *Pharmacotherapy*, *23*(1), 113–132. https://doi.org/10.1592/phco.23.1.113.31910

Talon, B., Perez, A., Yan, C., Alobaidi, A., Zhang, K. H., Schultz, B. G., Suda, K. J., & Touchette, D. R. (2019, December 27). Economic evaluations of clinical pharmacy services in the United States: 2011-2017. *JACCP: JOURNAL OF THE AMERICAN COLLEGE OF CLINICAL PHARMACY*, *3*(4), 793–806. https://doi.org/10.1002/jac5.1199

Terris-Prestholt, F., Quaife, M., & Vickerman, P. (2016, January 15). Parameterising User Uptake in Economic Evaluations: The role of discrete choice experiments. *Health Economics*, *25*, 116–123. https://doi.org/10.1002/hec.3297

Touchette, D. R., Doloresco, F., Suda, K. J., Perez, A., Turner, S., Jalundhwala, Y., Tangonan, M. C., & Hoffman, J. M. (2014, March 19). Economic Evaluations of Clinical Pharmacy Services: 2006-2010. *Pharmacotherapy: The Journal of Human Pharmacology and Drug Therapy*, *34*(8), 771–793. https://doi.org/10.1002/phar.1414

Vanagas, G., Bala, M., & Lhachimi, S. K. (2017). Evidence-Based Public Health 2017. *BioMed Research International*, *2017*, 1–2. https://doi.org/10.1155/2017/2607397

van Mastrigt, G. A., Hiligsmann, M., Arts, J. J., Broos, P. H., Kleijnen, J., Evers, S. M., & Majoie, M. H. (2016, November 1). How to prepare a systematic review of economic evaluations for informing evidence-based healthcare decisions: a five-step approach (part 1/3). *Expert Review of Pharmacoeconomics & Outcomes Research*, *16*(6), 689–704. https://doi.org/10.1080/14737167.2016.1246960

YOUR KNOWLEDGE HAS VALUE

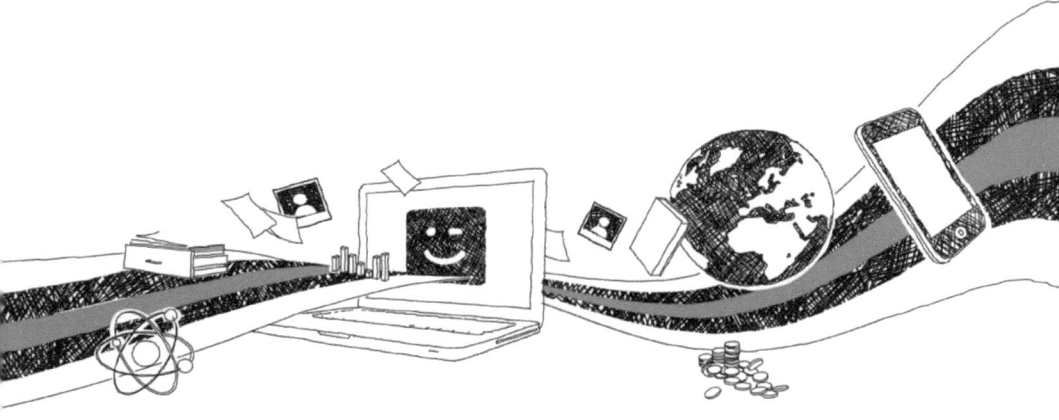

- We will publish your bachelor's and
  master's thesis, essays and papers

- Your own eBook and book -
  sold worldwide in all relevant shops

- Earn money with each sale

Upload your text at www.GRIN.com
and publish for free

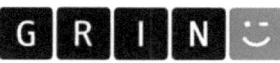

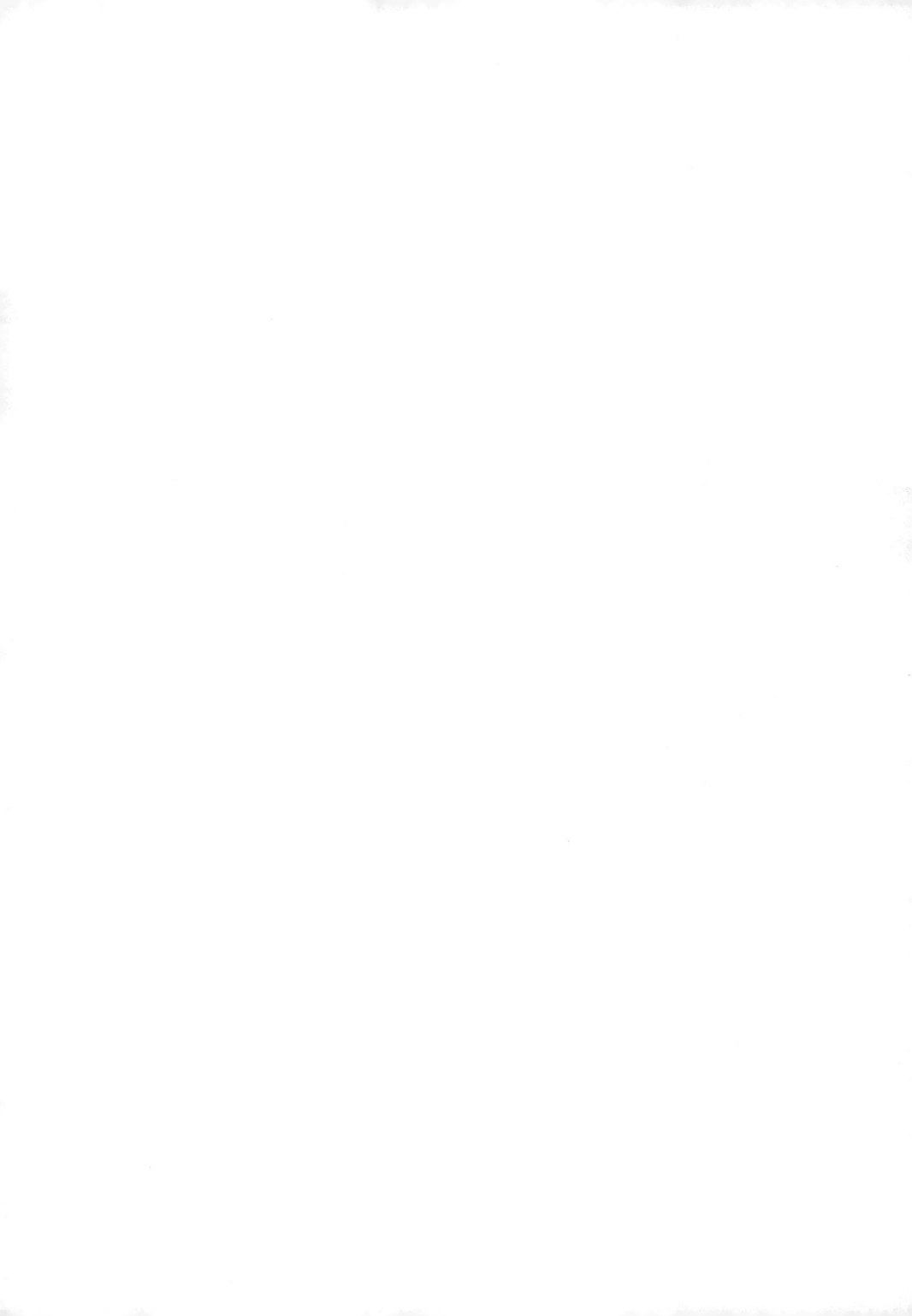